Introduction

I love hill walking. Although I enjoy the challenge of the climb, for me it's the prize waiting at the top that spurs me on... that breathtaking, indescribably beautiful view as creation stretches beneath your feet and further than your eye can see.

Several essentials, however, are required before heading out, a map or guide book being the most important. The best of these not only head you in the right direction but highlight viewing points, steep gradients and potential hazards along the way. Other essentials include great company, plasters, chocolate (plenty), water, waterproofs (!) and a celebratory picnic for the top.

The journey through the menopause can, for some, be like a mountain climb whilst for others it's as easy as a walk in the park. But for all women, the menopause marks a significant change in life which can have consequences on long-term health, emotions and relationships.

My hope is that this book enables you to more easily understand the medicine of the menopause, its signs, symptoms and treatments, that it equips you to deal with the longer-term effects on your health and relationships and serves as a step by step 'survival guide' to getting you through the uphill climb so you can truly say... 'the view is good from here'.

About The Author

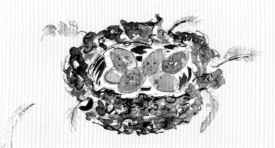

Lou has been a GP in Suffolk, specialising in women's medicine, for over 15 years. She now also works as a GP tutor at Cambridge University Clinical School helping lead seminars on Ethics and the Law. She lives with her husband, Robert, their adorable Westie dog Lily and Alice, a very beautiful but headstrong cat.

Contents...

Keeping Your Cool In The Heat Of The Night

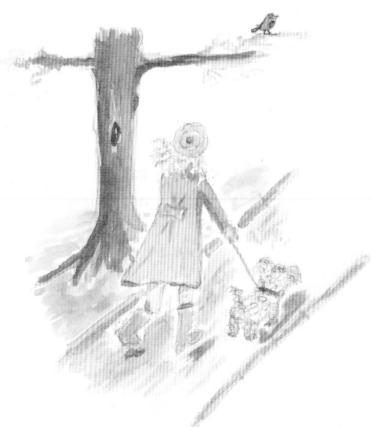

A Survival Guide To The Menopause

Written And Illustrated By
Dr Lou Cowan MB, BS, DRCOG

Robin House Books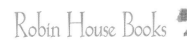

For:

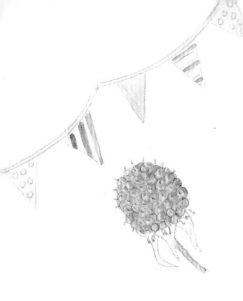

Robert ~
who holds my hand and has
my heart. Come fly with me......
And for Jane ~
my sister and best friend.
With special thanks to my mum and (late)
dad who saw me through medical school and
so made this possible.

With Thanks:

It is such a privilege to have this opportunity to thank people in words that will not fade
with the passage of time. Firstly, thank you to my gorgeous husband Robert, for your endless
love and support. Here's a book about flying! Thank you to my wonderful family and friends,
too many to name individually but you know who you are. Thank you for believing in me,
standing with me and brushing me down when I fall. For cheering me on through the
thicks and thins of life with your love, prayers, laughter and encouragement. It is an
honour to know you and my thanks to you stretch wider than any ocean.
Sally, Janie, Mary and Caroline thank you for proof reading this book, for your
tremendous encouragement, insight and friendship. Thanks for pointing me in the
right direction! Jill, for all your love, friendship and support, thank you.
Charlotte, it's been a joy working with you in the design of this book. Thank you for your
patience, understanding and friendship. I hope you go from strength to strength!
Thank you to all my amazing friends at Kingsgate... may your wells be deep and overflowing.
And finally, thank you to my heavenly Father, who makes all things possible and who gently
holds me in His hand. To Him I owe everything.
Lou x

Chapter One

What Is The Menopause And Why Does It Happen?

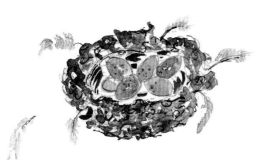

Some Definitions:

The 'menopause' is officially diagnosed when a woman has been free from any periods or menstrual bleeds for at least 12 months; in essence the menopause is her final period and is caused by irreversible changes in female hormones that may be verified by blood tests if the diagnosis is uncertain.

MARCH

A YEAR ON FROM THE LAST PERIOD

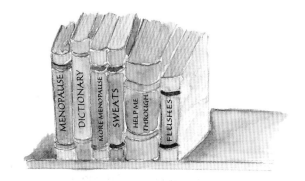

MENOPAUSE
DICTIONARY
MORE MENOPAUSE
SWEATS
HELP ME THROUGH
FLUSHES

It is sometimes referred to as 'the change' and marks the ending of a woman's fertile years, although contraception may still be required (see page 8).

THIS TIME OF LIFE CAN BE AN EMOTIONAL ROLLERCOASTER...

The 'perimenopause' (sometimes called the 'climacteric') is the time leading up to the menopause, during which periods may well be irregular, or other symptoms, such as hot flushes or emotional changes, experienced... it may go on for years.

OFF TO THE SUN!

This is not the winter of your life; it's a new season.

The 'postmenopause' is the time following the menopause.

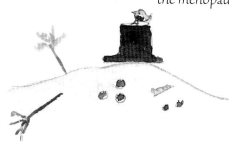

In Britain, the average age for the menopause is 51... but for many women, their periods stop in their forties.

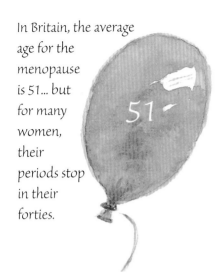

Some women under the age of 45 may have an early or 'premature' menopause. It is estimated that premature menopause affects 1% of women under the age of 40 and 0.1% under the age of 30. This can be a very difficult diagnosis for a woman to handle, especially if she has not had a family. Treatment and counselling should be given in all such cases (see 'special cases' on page 5 and page 32).

THIS IS A UNIQUE SEASON OF YOUR LIFE, ONE TO EMBRACE WITH ITS RICH AND VARIED COLOURS

Around 80% of women in the UK have noticeable symptoms, hot flushes and night sweats being two of the most common.

Millions of women, all over the world, enter the menopause every year. It is not a disease but it may have consequences on your health and your quality of life, so...

A LITTLE READING AROUND THE SUBJECT GOES A LONG WAY.

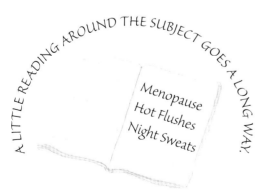

Menopause
Hot Flushes
Night Sweats

A blood test may be required for these younger women, to distinguish between the menopause and other causes of total lack of periods (amenorrhoea). These include pregnancy, extreme weight loss, excessive exercise, thyroid problems, certain medications and surgery, to mention but a few!

What Causes The Menopause?

We are born with several million potential eggs, divided into 2 ovaries. Only a fraction of these develop and mature.

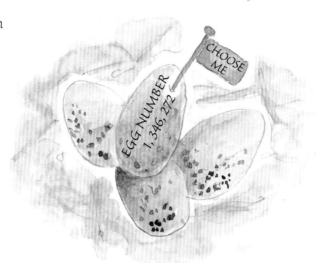

When we start our periods, usually in the early teens, we become fertile. One egg (sometimes more) matures and is released into the womb. This usually happens regularly every month and is controlled by several hormones – the two most well known are Oestrogen and Progesterone. If the egg is not fertilised, a decrease in progesterone levels cause a menstrual bleed or period and the cycle starts all over again.

Two other hormones, Follicle Stimulating Hormone (FSH) and Luteinising Hormone (LH), are also intricately linked to egg production and release. The closer to the menopause you get, the higher the FSH becomes. It is the change in the levels of these two hormones that can be assessed, by blood tests, which may help diagnose the menopause. Symptoms, however, are usually the best diagnosis.

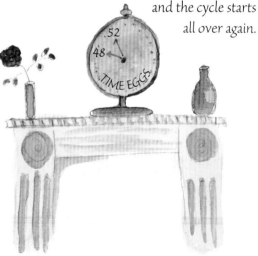

Usually, at around the age of 50, the last egg is released.

In the years immediately preceding the menopause (the perimenopause) periods may become very irregular as hormone levels start to alter. Eggs may not be released every cycle... and physical and emotional symptoms, indicating the approach of the menopause, may occur.

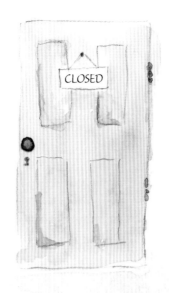

After 12 months of no periods or cycles, the menopause can be officially diagnosed. Occasionally the diagnosis can be uncertain or a sudden bleed may occur after 12 months of being period-free. Further investigation by your doctor will be required if this is the case.

Eventually, no matter how hard our hormones push to release another egg from the ovaries, allowing either for fertilisation or a period, no further eggs are available. Because of this, oestrogen and progesterone levels drop, and this causes the menopause to occur.

Special Cases

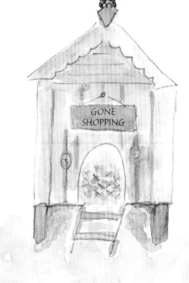

As mentioned earlier, for some, the menopause can arrive unexpectedly at a much earlier age or be brought on due to medication, such as chemotherapy, or surgical removal of the ovaries (oophorectomy). This can be a very difficult diagnosis, particularly if the woman hasn't had a family. Specialist counselling and support is available in such cases.

For women who go through the menopause before the age of 45, it is important that HRT is prescribed until around the age of a natural average menopause (51). This helps protect against osteoporosis and heart disease.

THIS IS A SEASON OF NEW BEGINNINGS

THERE IS HOPE FOR YOUR FUTURE

Chapter Two

What Are The Signs And Symptoms Of The Menopause?

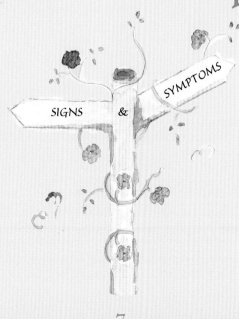

Symptoms

The effects of the menopause can be divided into
~ Early Symptoms and
~ Late or Longer-term Symptoms
They can also be divided into
~ Physical and
~ Emotional Symptoms...

PHYSICAL SYMPTOMS

HOT FLUSHES... MOOD SWINGS...
NIGHT SWEATS...

EMOTIONAL SYMPTOMS

TO HELP UNRAVEL THESE, LET'S LOOK AT THE MOST COMMON...

Many women have few symptoms and will sail through the menopausal years with ease; for others, however, this uncharted territory is a far rockier ride, with many uphill struggles and downhill emotions. Such emotions can mimic, or coincide with, depression, making this a difficult time for you and your nearest and dearest.

IRREGULAR CYCLES

Most women enter the 'perimenopause' (the lead up to the menopause) in their 40s. One of the first tell-tale signs of this is that monthly cycles or periods become irregular and/or sometimes heavier or longer.

PREGNANCY TEST

The gap in-between periods may become longer or shorter or periods may be missed for months at a time... BUT PLEASE REMEMBER... you are still fertile during this time and need to use contraception for at least 2 further years if your last period (menopause) is before the age of 50, or for 1 year if your last period is at the age of 50 or over.

Early Symptoms

~Physical Symptoms~ the most common include hot flushes, night sweats, painful sex, dry and itchy skin, poor sleep, headaches/migraines, palpitations, aches and pains, dry hair and dry eyes and skin. All these symptoms are largely due to a drop in oestrogen.

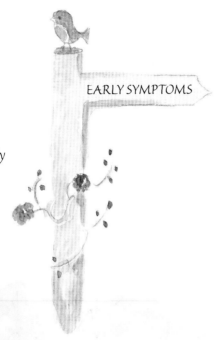

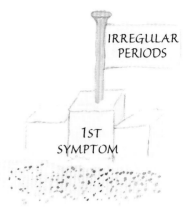

But don't despair, help is at hand. Being forewarned about possible symptoms is most definitely forearmed. So please read on...

Emotional Symptoms

~ the most common include mood swings, irritability, anxiety, poor concentration and memory lapses (made far worse by lack of sleep), fatigue, loss of interest in sex, loss of confidence and poor self-esteem.

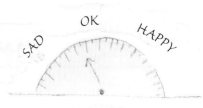

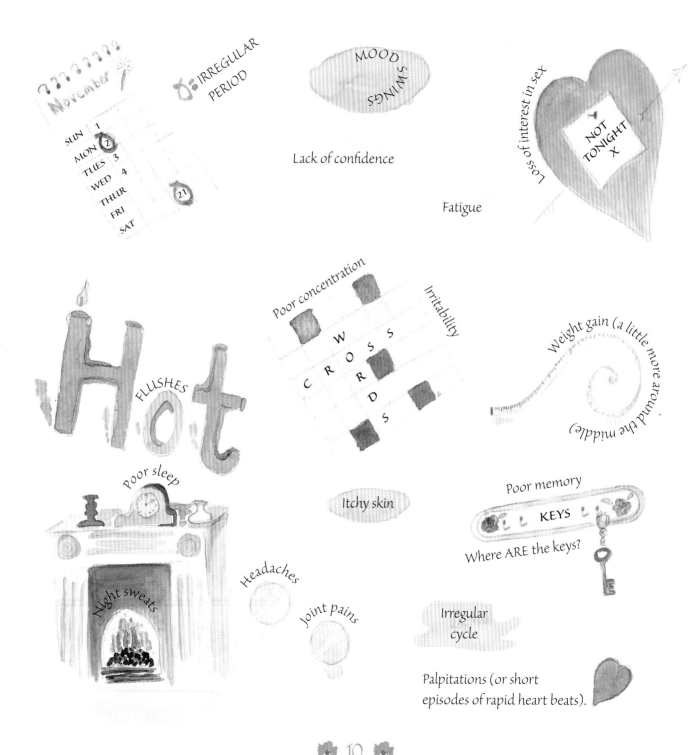

November

SUN 1
MON 2
TUES 3
WED 4
THUR
FRI
SAT
21

IRREGULAR PERIOD

MOOD SWINGS

Lack of confidence

Loss of interest in sex

NOT TONIGHT X

Fatigue

Poor concentration

CROSS WORDS

Irritability

Weight gain (a little more around the middle)

Hot FLUSHES

Poor sleep

Itchy skin

Poor memory

KEYS

Where ARE the keys?

Night sweats

Headaches

Joint pains

Irregular cycle

Palpitations (or short episodes of rapid heart beats).

Later Symptoms

These can be divided into three main areas:
~Osteoporosis~ so important a whole chapter has been dedicated to it.
~Heart disease~
~Urogenital Atrophy~ what's that? In other words, the effect of the menopause on the bladder and vaginal regions causing...

vaginal dryness
vaginal itching or burning
painful sex
cystitis (urine infections)
incontinence

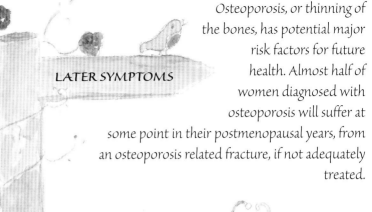

LATER SYMPTOMS

Osteoporosis, or thinning of the bones, has potential major risk factors for future health. Almost half of women diagnosed with osteoporosis will suffer at some point in their postmenopausal years, from an osteoporosis related fracture, if not adequately treated.

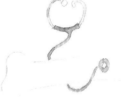

Don't despair! There are things you can start doing now which will effectively help and improve the future health of your bones, heart and urogenital area. To find out how, please read on...

The Heart of the Matter...

The oestrogen we produce before the menopause also has a protective effect on our heart... so after the menopause women are far more at risk of heart disease, including angina and heart attacks. In fact, sadly and possibly surprisingly, heart disease is the most common cause of death in women over the age of 60...
second commonest being a stroke...
the third being breast cancer.
So, there's no time like the present to start looking at how to improve your health and lower your risks.

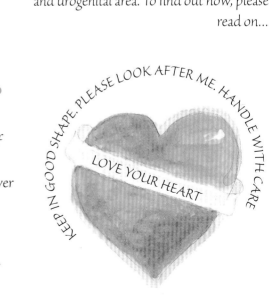

KEEP IN GOOD SHAPE. PLEASE LOOK AFTER ME. HANDLE WITH CARE

LOVE YOUR HEART

The major risk factors of heart disease in women are…
smoking, raised cholesterol, raised blood pressure (hypertension), lack of exercise, a
family history of heart disease, diabetes, previous
stroke or mini stroke (TIA) and increasing age
(not too much you can do about this one). Also
if your BMI (Body Mass Index) classifies you as
'obese' and your waist circumference is more than 88cm, your risk of heart disease is
significantly increased.
So please, if you have any of the risk factors of heart disease or feel that your heart
health isn't what it should be, do visit your GP or the practice nurse to chat it over.
Be aware of your heart so it can wear well for you.

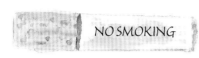

NO SMOKING

EAT WELL

Don't Be Shy…

NO SEX (OR INCONTINENCE) PLEASE… WE'RE BRITISH

Now what about the effect of the menopause on your
bladder, vaginal region and your sex life? These can be the
hardest of symptoms to talk about and hence thousands
of women, every year, suffer in silence and go untreated.
Most, if not all women, will experience one or more of
the following:
vaginal dryness, painful sex, vaginal itching or burning,
urinary incontinence and urine infections.

Such symptoms are due to declining
oestrogen around the bladder and vagina.
This can lead to potentially quite profound physical and
therefore psychological and emotional symptoms. Don't
despair, help is at hand…

 12

Local oestrogen creams can help enormously with vaginal symptoms (see page 23 on local HRT). The majority of women find great relief after a few weeks of use. Incontinence and urinary infections (cystitis) can be treated with a range of short or long-term treatments. Pelvic floor exercises, if done regularly, can also help some women. However, at times, incontinence can so affect a woman's day to day life and thus her self-esteem that an operation (usually highly effective) may be required. So don't keep your symptoms locked away. Take courage and ask for help, it's available for you.

OESTROGEN CREAM

DON'T KEEP YOUR SYMPTOMS LOCKED AWAY

COMMUNICATION IS THE NAME OF THE GAME

Remember to talk to your nearest and dearest about how you are feeling, particularly if your love life is dwindling. It's hard for them to understand, especially when you lock your feelings away. Communication can help keep your relationship strong and healthy.

In Summary:

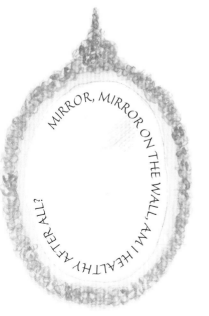

MIRROR, MIRROR ON THE WALL, AM I HEALTHY AFTER ALL?

Around 80% of women will have one or more noticeable or distressing symptoms of hormonal changes in the months or years leading up to the menopause and beyond, the most usual being irregular periods, hot flushes and emotional swings. Officially, the menopause is your last period and so can only really be diagnosed retrospectively.

The menopause is an excellent time in life to reassess your general health, diet and fitness.

Put time and effort into protecting your heart, bones and relationships! If symptoms persist, are distressing or worrying, take courage and see your doctor, who is very likely to have helped many women through the menopause.

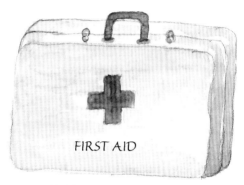

FIRST AID

HELP IS ON THE WAY

Chapter Three

The Emotions Of The Menopause For You And Yours

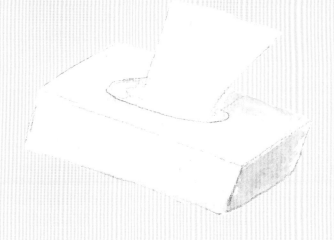

Emotional Changes

The menopausal years can be an incredibly difficult time for many women. Hormonal changes may cause huge emotional downs similar to, or even mistaken for, depression. On top of this, changes in body shape, loss of libido, a poor sleep pattern and anxiety can cause confidence to drop and self-esteem to tumble.

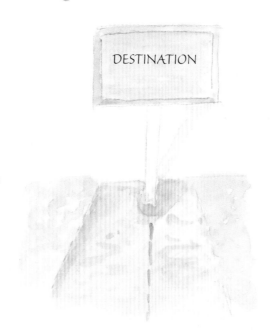

DESTINATION

But don't despair, your wings are not clipped and you will fly again.

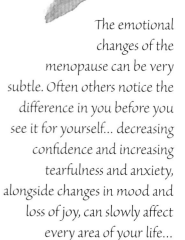

The emotional changes of the menopause can be very subtle. Often others notice the difference in you before you see it for yourself... decreasing confidence and increasing tearfulness and anxiety, alongside changes in mood and loss of joy, can slowly affect every area of your life...

...but knowing this is a natural process and that the hormonal imbalances which caused it will settle down (and can be treated) brings hope and a light at the end of the tunnel.

It is very important that you care for and make time for yourself. It is also essential that you communicate with your nearest and dearest about how you are feeling. It may not be easy for your household either, as hormonal changes and the unstable emotions that they can bring may be difficult to understand or live with. This chapter is especially for your loved ones. Hope it helps!

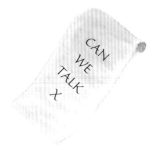

CAN WE TALK x

For You...

Why not try learning something new or join a book club or a gym class... find a walking group or get an allotment!

'Treats' Menu
~Spend quality time with your nearest and dearest.
~Book a free makeover with a department store.
~Settle down with a good book or a chick flick.
~Have coffee or lunch out with an understanding friend (take some tissues).
~Both laughter and tears can be very therapeutic!
~Get plenty of fresh air and exercise.
~Enjoy a long bath.
~Get a dog (optional). They are always happy to see you! X

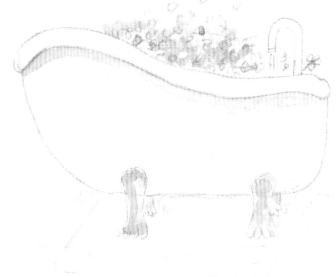

If you forget most of the information you've just read (and memory loss can be a very frustrating symptom) try to remember and hold on to these three points...

1) You will get through this difficult time. Changes in emotions and the physical symptoms which can accompany the menopause will settle down over time.

2) Communicate (gently) with your loved ones. It's hard for them too.

3) Love and look after yourself. You're worth it!

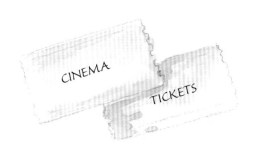

CINEMA TICKETS

A Little Note For Your Nearest And Dearest For Him...

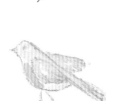

If you have a man in your life, please ask him (nicely) to read this...
The menopause can be an incredibly difficult time, both emotionally and physically, for the woman in your life. The hormones and 'monthly cycle' that she has relied upon for many years (and that you probably have a healthy respect for) start to spiral out of control. This causes mood swings and sometimes quite irrational behaviour. You may also notice other changes in her such as...
ANXIETY, LOW MOOD, TEARFULNESS, LOW SEX DRIVE (you're likely to spot this one early!) IRRITABILITY, MEMORY LAPSES, WEIGHT GAIN, POOR SELF-ESTEEM and more.
For the sake of your relationship, please be understanding. Try to listen to her, and, more importantly, love her, through all these changes.

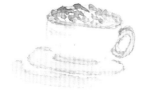

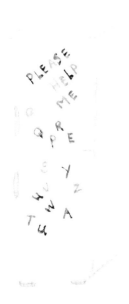

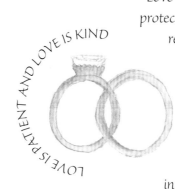

Love is patient and kind. This is a time to build and protect your relationship. It can be a time of growth, renewed communication and commitment. It's a good time for positive planning. Invest in your future together. Learn or re-learn to love each other and to understand how the other 'ticks'. Sometimes all she needs is a hug or a compliment to help see her through a difficult day. How about booking in some time for just the two of you each week? Spending quality time together doesn't have to be expensive.

To The Kids...

Okay, so your mum may be constantly hormonal, generally acting a bit weird and blaming you for... well just about everything... but remember, she is still your mum, and let's face it, you can be pretty emotional too!

So here are some helpful hints on how to deal with your mum when she's being really irrational...

Try giving her... a hug, her favourite meal, a wide berth or at least some space! A compliment, a bunch of flowers, less of your lip and more of your love, a quiet night in, a lovely night out. This is a hard time for your mum and not great for you either, but try to love her through it.

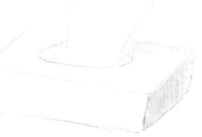

THE KIDS

For Your Best Friend...

Be there for her, as you always are. Try not to become defensive if she is irritable or emotional. Give her a listening ear and plenty of tissues. It's likely you can relate to some of these hormonal changes, or will do soon.

BEST FRIEND

LOVE IS SLOW TO BECOME ANGRY BUT QUICK TO FORGIVE

PS... For Your Other Best Friend ...

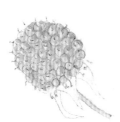

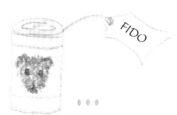

FIDO

JUST KEEP WAGGING THAT TAIL OR PURRING THAT PURR, WASH THE DISHES (NO LICKING!)

DOG

CAT

AND CLEAN UP AFTER YOURSELF. OFFER TO MAKE SUPPER…OR MAYBE NOT

Chapter Four

The Question Of HRT

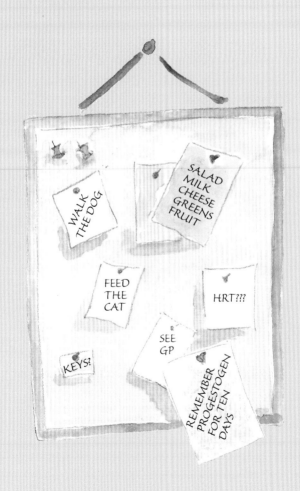

A Change In Season For Hormone Replacement Therapy

Hormone replacement therapy, or 'HRT', has caused a great deal of debate, concern and confusion over the past decade. This has thrown most women and their GPs into questioning its safety... We are not amused and we are very confused... heads or tails, should we use it or not?

WE ARE NOT AMUSED AND WE ARE VERY CONFUSED...

Actually, the worries about prescribing HRT have virtually turned full circle since 2001 as new data (and reviews of old trials) have confirmed HRT as the most effective and beneficial treatment for short and long-term symptoms of the menopause.

WELL DONE!

1ST

GOOD SHOW!.

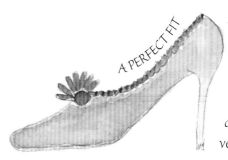

A PERFECT FIT

Symptoms such as... hot flushes, night sweats, low sex drive (low libido), aches and pains, painful intercourse, anxiety, itchy skin, urinary symptoms, depression and irritability... can all be very effectively treated with the right dosage and formulation of HRT to suit the needs of most individuals.

The Right HRT For Your Individual Needs...

HRT can either be given

~Systemically (reaching all areas of the body) ~ by oral route (mouth), using tablets, or a
  non-oral route, using patches, sprays or even gels...

Or

~Locally (targeting a particular area of the body) ~ most commonly via oestrogen around
  the vaginal region or measured dosages of oestrogen into the vagina via a pessary. It can
  even be given via a flexible ring, containing oestrogen, which is inserted into
  the vagina and changed every 3 months.

HRT can either be

~Combined ~ containing both oestrogen and progestogen (a synthetic form of the
  natural hormone progesterone). Progestogen is required to protect the lining
  of the womb (see below).

Or

~Oestrogen only ~ for women who have had a hysterectomy (removal of the womb) or for
  any woman where just 'local' treatment is preferred or required.

Oestrogen and progestogen MUST be taken together in those women who still have a womb.
Progestogen balances the potentially harmful effects that oestrogen-only treatment can cause to
the womb lining. Without progestogen, these changes could eventually lead to cancer
of the womb... oestrogen with progestogen creates the perfect balance.

Progestogens are given either as oral tablets or combined with oestrogen in a patch. They can also
be given via the Mirena coil, where a small dose of progestogen is released daily into the womb.
Many women opt for the coil as it also offers effective contraception around the
peri-menopause and early menopause years. HRT itself is NOT a contraceptive.

If you start HRT when you are still having periods, (before the menopause), you will
need to take it on a monthly cycle and therefore still have bleeds...
However, if you haven't had a period for over a year (officially in the menopause) you can take
HRT continuously, no cycle and no bleed.

Confused? You won't be. Turn the page and see the HRT Decision Tree...

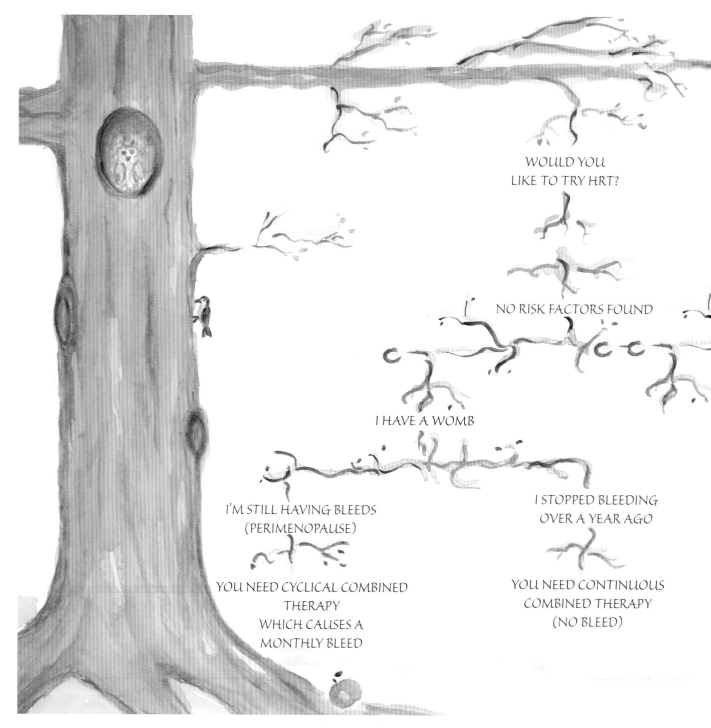

WOULD YOU
LIKE TO TRY HRT?

NO RISK FACTORS FOUND

I HAVE A WOMB

I'M STILL HAVING BLEEDS
(PERIMENOPAUSE)

YOU NEED CYCLICAL COMBINED
THERAPY
WHICH CAUSES A
MONTHLY BLEED

I STOPPED BLEEDING
OVER A YEAR AGO

YOU NEED CONTINUOUS
COMBINED THERAPY
(NO BLEED)

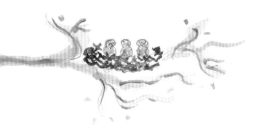

The HRT Decision Tree...

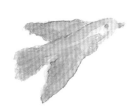

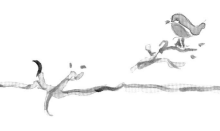

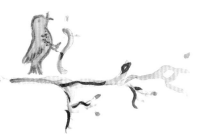

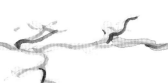

I'VE HAD A
HYSTERECTOMY

I STILL HAVE A WOMB BUT
I ONLY NEED TREATMENT
FOR MY BLADDER AND/OR
VAGINA

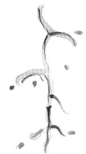

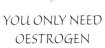

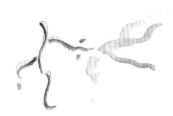

YOU ONLY NEED
OESTROGEN

YOU ONLY NEED LOCAL OR
TOPICAL OESTROGEN

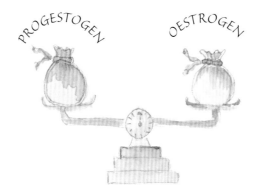

PERFECTLY BALANCED IN HRT TO
PROTECT THE WOMB LINING

Chapter Five

HRT...
Is It For Me?

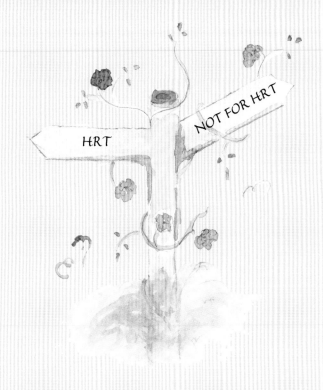

The Good, The Bad And The Ugly

Although HRT can be very beneficial, it may not be for you. As with all medication there are... SIDE EFFECTS, RISKS and CONTRAINDICATIONS. So do you have the 'all clear' or is HRT the wrong choice for you?

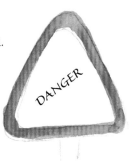

DANGER

The Committee on Safety of Medicines (CSM) and the British National Formulary (BNF) have given clear guidelines for prescribing HRT, which state that...

HRT is an effective relief for menopausal symptoms. When the benefits of prescribing outweigh the risks, the lowest effective dose should be used for a short duration of up to 5 years. Sometimes it is required for longer. The need for HRT should be assessed, with a check-up, on at least an annual basis. When deciding to stop HRT, it should be phased out slowly.

SOME OF THE COMMONEST SIDE EFFECTS OF HRT INCLUDE...

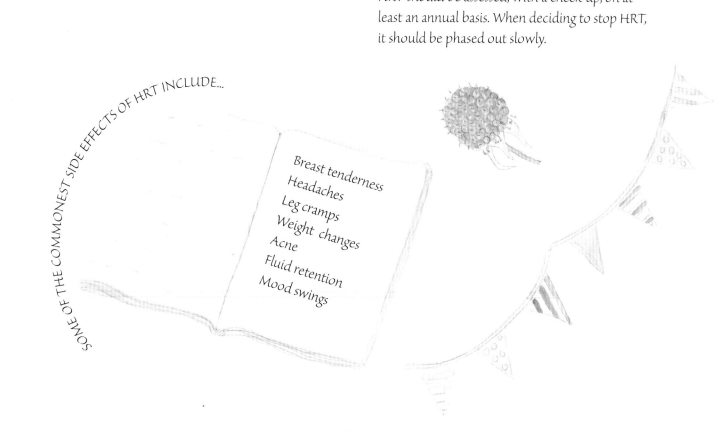

Breast tenderness
Headaches
Leg cramps
Weight changes
Acne
Fluid retention
Mood swings

Short-Term Benefits

Some of the benefits of taking HRT may be felt very quickly... confidence returns and emotional ups and downs start to level out. Hot flushes and night sweats improve rapidly. Loss of libido (sex drive) tends to improve as do generalised aches and pains.

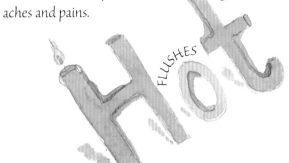

Longer-Term Benefits

Reduction or prevention of osteoporosis and of the symptoms of arthritis...an added 'boneness' (sorry!). Reduction in the risk of bowel cancer. New evidence suggests that HRT may reduce the risk and onset of dementia. If started on or around the menopause and before the age of 60, HRT may protect from heart disease.

What About The Side Effects?

Any medication has the potential to cause side effects. HRT is no exception to this rule. Common side effects include... mood swings, breast tenderness and enlargement, headaches, leg cramps, pre-menstrual tension, acne and fluid retention. It is also common to experience spotting or irregular bleeding when starting HRT. However, if this continues for 6 months or more after the start of treatment, it is important that you are assessed by your GP. Around a third of women stop taking HRT because of side effects, although just changing the dose or type of HRT often helps.

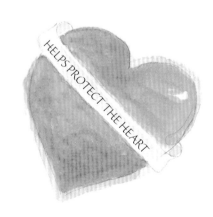

HELPS PROTECT THE HEART

Those That Should Be Cautious...

Check with your doctor before starting HRT, particularly if you have previously been diagnosed with breast lumps, endometriosis, fibroids or gallstones. These can sometimes be made worse by taking HRT.

For some, HRT is absolutely contraindicated (contraindications are reasons you can never take it). You will need to discuss other options for treatment with your GP or local specialist clinic if you have any of the following...

> Past or current breast cancer
> Undiagnosed breast lump(s)
> Family history of breast cancer
> Other current cancer
> Undiagnosed abnormal bleeding
> Liver disease
> Active heart disease
> Deep vein thrombosis (DVT)

FOR SOME, THE DOOR TO HRT IS...

CLOSED

I'M WORRIED. CAN YOU GIVE ME SOME ADVICE?

There are other, less common, contraindications to taking HRT; it's always worth getting advice. Of course, if you have started HRT and you get symptoms such as severe chest pain, leg pain (especially in the calf), shortness of breath or severe abdominal pain, you need to seek advice URGENTLY.

What Are The Risks Of Taking HRT?

The most important risks associated with HRT use are ~

    Breast cancer

    Blood clots in the veins (venous thrombosis)

    Blood clots in the arteries (arterial thrombosis),

  which may lead to heart attacks and/or strokes

    Cancer of the lining of the womb

HOWEVER it is always important to put risks into perspective, remembering that most women on HRT experience no such problems... in fact, it appears that SMOKING, EXCESSIVE ALCOHOL intake and OBESITY are more likely to put women at risk of breast cancer and blood clots!

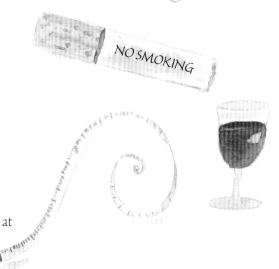

HRT And Breast Cancer ~ Unravelling The Risk

Many women have been put off choosing HRT to help with menopausal symptoms, because of the link it has with increasing their risk of breast cancer. But just how big a risk is it?

Sadly, breast cancer is one of the most significant and devastating of illnesses of the Western world. Most of us know someone deeply affected by this disease. Being 'breast aware' is strongly promoted in our society and excellent campaigns, research and screening programmes (using mammograms or ultrasound scans) are continually helping in the battle against it... breast cancer is always in the news...

HRT has had a great deal of bad press, due to its links with breast cancer, but is it all true?

Studies in the last decade have certainly shown an association between HRT (especially with the 'combined' form of oestrogen and progestogen) and certain types of breast cancer. However, statistically the risks appear to be small and strongly linked with the duration of therapy. But what does this actually mean for you? Here are some relatively simple statistics (maths was never my strong point) to put the risk into perspective...

~ A 50 year old woman who has never taken and never will take HRT has around a 4.5% risk of developing breast cancer by the time she is 70.
~ A 50 year old woman who takes combined HRT (oestrogen and progestogen) for 5 years has around a 4.8% risk of developing breast cancer by the time she is 70.
~ A 50 year old woman who takes combined HRT for 10 years has around a 5.4% risk of developing breast cancer by the time she is 70. Summarised from medical publishings.

Therefore, a short duration of combined HRT, 5 years or less, is thought to give effective relief of menopausal symptoms with little increase in risk of breast cancer.
10 years of combined HRT increases the risk of breast cancer significantly.
So the 5 year rule is a good one to follow, although some women may want HRT for longer. The benefits and risks of this can be discussed with your GP.
Remember to have an annual check-up for your HRT, no matter how busy you are or how well you feel!

A special note for those diagnosed with an early (under 45) or premature (under 40) menopause...taking HRT up until the time of the average age of natural menopause does NOT appear to increase the risk of breast cancer, heart disease or a stroke.

Other Risks Of Using HRT Include...

~A slightly increased risk of developing ovarian cancer. This is linked to long-term use of
  either combined or oestrogen only HRT.
~A slightly increased risk of developing a deep vein thrombosis (DVT) or pulmonary
  embolism (PE). The risk seems to decrease after the first year of use. However, severe
  varicose veins and obesity can also increase your risk of a DVT or PE, as can prolonged
  bed rest, such as that required after surgery. So in such cases HRT may not be
  appropriate for you, or may have to be stopped. It is worth noting that using
  the HRT patch may eliminate this increased risk of DVT and PE.
~Womb cancer. Remember to protect your womb from any potential increase
  in risk of cancer. A progestogen must be taken for 10 to 14 days of every 28 day cycle,
  when using combined, systemic form of HRT... your doctor knows this, but it's good to
  have this information at your fingertips.

Stopping HRT

On average, women take HRT for about 2 years. When the time comes, it is best to stop it gradually over 3-6 months, by
slowly reducing the dose. Stopping suddenly may cause some symptoms to return.
For some women, especially those whose mothers suffered severe symptoms of flushes and sweats, coming off HRT can be
extremely difficult. The return of symptoms may force them to go back onto HRT longer-term. This is a very personal choice
and one to be discussed with your GP.

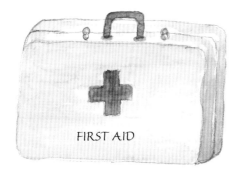

FIRST AID

In Summary...

HRT is a very effective treatment for reducing or relieving many of the
symptoms of the menopause, as well as helping reduce some of the long-
term consequences that the menopausal years can bring. It does have some
potential risks, but equally many potential benefits. These risks and benefits
need to be weighed up individually and with your GP, so that you can make
the right choice.

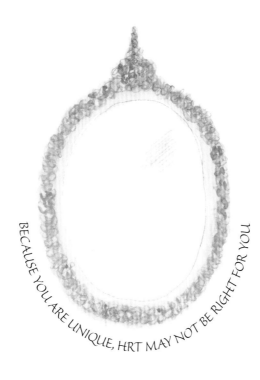

BECAUSE YOU ARE UNIQUE, HRT MAY NOT BE RIGHT FOR YOU

Chapter Six

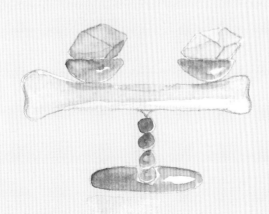

Osteoporosis
The 'Hole' Story

When at their prime, usually in our late 20s or early 30s, bones are a fantastically functional organ: a perfect balance between strength, density and weight...

MATURED TO PERFECTION

Our bones also have their own inbuilt mechanism for repairing, rebuilding and removing old bone. This is performed by two very clever types of cell, the osteoblasts and osteoclasts.

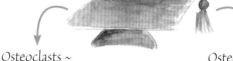

Osteoclasts ~
break down old bone

Osteoblasts ~
repair, rebuild and lay down new bone

Oestrogen is thought to help the activity of osteoblasts, hence a decline in oestrogen during and after the menopause causes the bone to be replaced less efficiently. So............. DENSITY DECREASES AND FRAGILITY INCREASES.

The word 'osteoporosis' is derived from Greek and literally means 'bones that have many holes', an apt description. Left alone, osteoporosis can lead to reduced bone density, deterioration of bone tissue and ultimately increased susceptibility to fractures.

A staggering one in every three women will have osteoporosis in the years following the menopause; roughly half of these women will suffer with an osteoporosis related fracture as they get older.
Some women are more at risk than others of developing osteoporosis and long-term medication may be required. However, every woman needs to put her best foot forward to ensure the healthiest future for her bones!

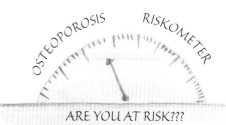

OSTEOPOROSIS RISKOMETER

ARE YOU AT RISK???

Because osteoporosis is strongly associated with fractures...
which can lead to chronic pain... and reduced mobility... and
potential loss of independence... it is essential that women at
risk are diagnosed early and treated appropriately.
Prevention is always better than cure.

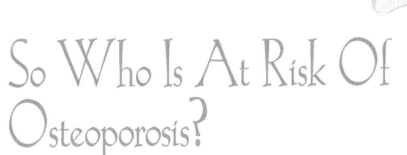

So Who Is At Risk Of Osteoporosis?

All women undergo bone loss around the menopause,
but some women are far more at risk of osteoporosis
than others. Are you at risk?

Low risk groups include ~

> No family history of osteoporosis
> Diet rich in calcium
> Plenty of weight-bearing
> exercise
> Early onset of periods
> Later menopause

Higher risk groups include ~

> Family history of osteoporosis
> The elderly
> Diabetics, smokers and heavy
> drinkers ~ another reason to
> stop smoking and take care of
> your diet
> Those diagnosed with an early
> menopause
> Those wheelchair or bed bound
> Long-term steroid users
> Anorexics past or present
> Coeliacs
> Inflammatory bowel disease
> sufferers

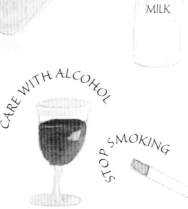

So In Summary

Bones love ~ calcium, exercise and
a good balanced diet.
Bones don't like ~ inactivity,
cigarettes (or dogs!).

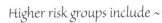

LOVE YOUR BONES

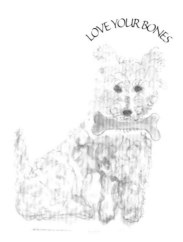

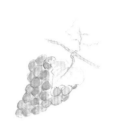

Chapter Seven

Diagnosing And Treating Osteoporosis

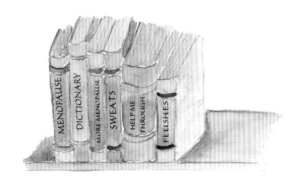

Osteoporosis, A Hidden Condition?

Some fractures can go completely unnoticed, with little or no pain. At other times, a minor fall or injury can cause a major fracture, leading to pain, immobility and even loss of independence.

Some women may find that each year they are getting a little shorter, or is it that everyone else is getting a little taller? Crush fractures of the vertebrae (spine) can cause loss of height and chronic back pain.

A LITTLE SHORTER EACH YEAR??

Screening For Osteoporosis

CRITERIA FOR DEXA SCAN INCLUDE

UNTREATED EARLY MENOPAUSE ☐

FAMILY HISTORY OF OSTEOPOROSIS ☐

WHEELCHAIR BOUND ☐

LONG TERM STEROIDS ☐

MINIMAL TRAUMA FRACTURE ☐

With over 200,000 osteoporosis-related fractures in the UK every year, there is great value in screening women (and men) most at risk.

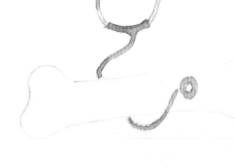

A bone mineral density X ray, or 'DEXA' scan, has been developed for such screening. Women who are considered to be 'at risk' are offered a scan and follow-up.

Are You At Risk Of Osteoporosis?

Because roughly HALF of women over the age of 50 with osteoporosis will have an osteoporosis-related fracture, it is vital that those most at risk are identified and treatment decisions made.

Calculating your own risk of osteoporosis is therefore very helpful and can now be done in the comfort of your own home via a new on-line risk calculator called FRAX. This clever questionnaire will calculate your likelihood, over the next 10 years, of a hip fracture or major osteoporotic fracture of the spine, shoulder or forearm. So being forewarned is potentially forearm protection!

TWITTER ABOUT IT

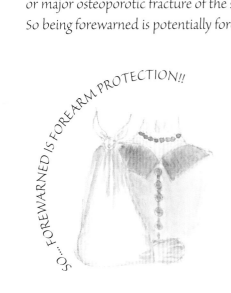

SO... FOREWARNED IS FOREARM PROTECTION!!

WHAT ELSE TAKES JUST 10 MINUTES...

ONE IN TWO ARE AT RISK...

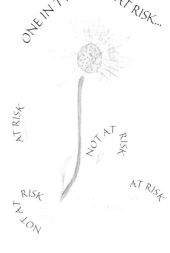

AT RISK

NOT AT RISK

NOT AT RISK

AT RISK

The FRAX score will also tell you whether you need to be referred for a bone mineral density X ray (DEXA scan) or whether you are at such high risk that you need to start treatment quickly. (See http://www.sheffield.ac.uk/FRAX/)
(what else takes just 10 minutes... running a bath, a quick jog, a cappuccino, try skimmed and decaf (skimmed because its low in fat and high in calcium, decaf because caffeine can make hot flushes worse... win-win), painting your nails, doing the weekly shopping – oh, if only!)

Minimising Your Risk And Maximising Bone Strength

As mentioned, bone density peaks around your early thirties, so a diet rich in calcium and plenty of weight-bearing exercise (especially before this age) will put your bones in excellent stead and will already have lessened your risk of osteoporosis...

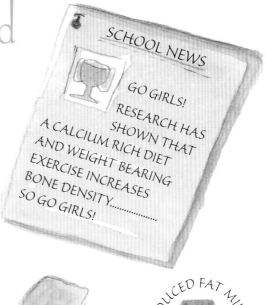

However, if you were never picked for the netball team or hid behind a tree instead of running cross-country at school, don't worry; you can start loving your bones today.

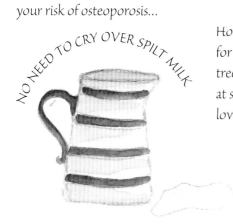

NO NEED TO CRY OVER SPILT MILK

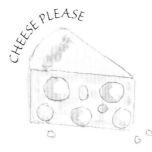

CHEESE PLEASE

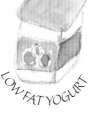

LOW FAT YOGURT

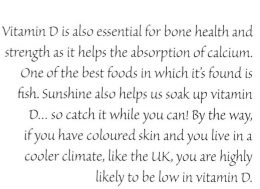

REDUCED FAT MILK

One of the easiest ways to love your bones is by increasing your calcium intake through dairy products such as ...cheese, milk and low fat yogurts (low fat or skimmed does not mean lower calcium). You can also take in calcium via tablet form if necessary.

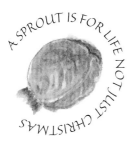

A SPROUT IS FOR LIFE NOT JUST CHRISTMAS

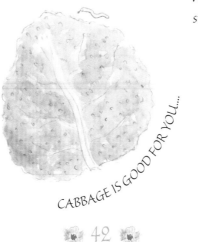

CABBAGE IS GOOD FOR YOU...

Vitamin D is also essential for bone health and strength as it helps the absorption of calcium. One of the best foods in which it's found is fish. Sunshine also helps us soak up vitamin D... so catch it while you can! By the way, if you have coloured skin and you live in a cooler climate, like the UK, you are highly likely to be low in vitamin D. Vitamin K is also important for building healthy bone tissue. Green leafy vegetables are an excellent source.

Exercise...

Exercise is a fantastic way to help strengthen your bones, keep fit and shed some extra pounds... and it doesn't have to cost a thing. The good news is you don't have to join a gym or run: a brisk walk is one of the best forms of weight-bearing exercise you can do.

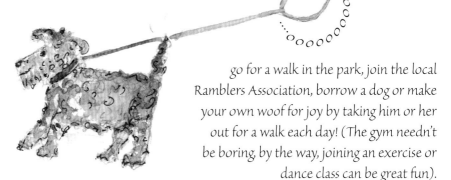

go for a walk in the park, join the local Ramblers Association, borrow a dog or make your own woof for joy by taking him or her out for a walk each day! (The gym needn't be boring, by the way, joining an exercise or dance class can be great fun).

At the end of the day, physical activity is helpful in maintaining your bone density and increasing muscle strength and fitness. Try building up your exercise to at least 30 minutes 3-4 times a week; you will feel all the better for it. But if your time is very constrained, skipping, hopscotch or even jumping up and down on the spot is better than nothing!

Medical Treatments Of Osteoporosis

Bisphosphonates and HRT are two of the most commonly prescribed treatments for osteoporosis and fracture prevention.
~HRT as mentioned in Chapter Five is very beneficial in protecting against post-menopausal osteoporosis, especially if started early in the menopause and taken for up to five years. However, HRT should not be used as the first-line treatment for osteoporosis.
~Bisphosphonates are an excellent way to treat osteoporosis. They reduce the breakdown of bone and can cut the risk of fractures by up to 50%. They can be taken daily, weekly or even once a month.
Remember to take your calcium tablets every day if needed.
Less commonly used treatments are also available, particularly for women who can't take either HRT or bisphosphonates. These include strontium ranelate, parathyroid hormone and Selective Oestrogen Receptor Modulators (SERMS for short).

In Summary: Love your bones and they will love you back!

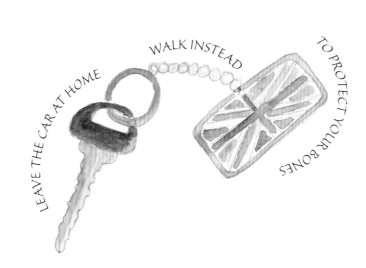

LEAVE THE CAR AT HOME WALK INSTEAD TO PROTECT YOUR BONES

Chapter Eight

Alternatives To HRT

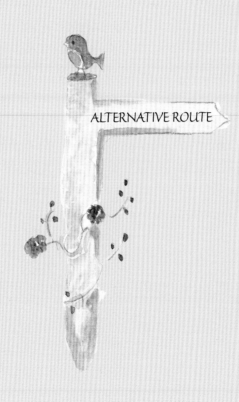

ALTERNATIVE ROUTE

No Thanks, HRT

For some women, HRT may be contraindicated and therefore too dangerous to take. See Chapter 5 for these contraindications. For many side effects or they want to try. may need to be the distressing of the others HRT may cause too may just not be a route Therefore alternatives found to help with symptoms menopause.

Due to popular demand and previous fears about HRT, there has been a huge growth in the use of alternative or natural therapies. A wide range of choices are now available, many of which appear to be helpful in the relief of menopausal symptoms.

There is little scientific evidence however for the effectiveness of some of these over-the-counter remedies. More importantly, not all natural remedies are completely safe.

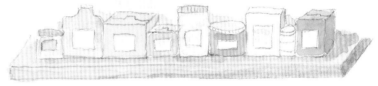

MENOPAUSE REMEDIES

Alternative Therapies

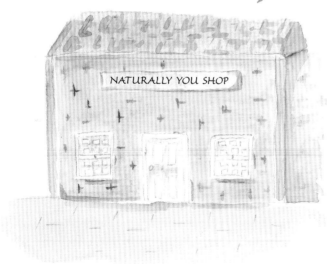

NATURALLY YOU SHOP

Prescribed alternatives to help with disturbing symptoms such as hot flushes include...

Clonidine~ usually given for high blood pressure or migraines. It may be of some benefit for a few women.

Progestogens~ a man-made form of progesterone, may help reduce flushes and sweats especially for women who cannot take HRT due to breast cancer. However, side-effects can outweigh benefits.

Selective Serotonin Reuptake Inhibitors (SSRIs) ~ normally used as antidepressants, can work well to reduce flushes and sweats. They are also helpful in controlling mood swings and some chronic pain conditions.

Gabapentin~ normally used to treat epilepsy, nerve pain or migraines, has been shown to help reduce hot flushes. However, side effects can limit its use.

Prescribed alternatives to HRT to help with osteoporosis, such as bisphosphonates, are dealt with in Chapter Seven.

Non-HRT vaginal moisturisers are available by prescription or over the counter, and can be beneficial in relieving vaginal dryness, vaginal discomfort and painful sex. Artificial lubricants coat the inside of the vagina and can continuously lubricate for a day or sometimes more; they can be applied well before intercourse.

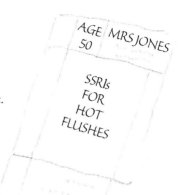

AGE MRS JONES
50

SSRIs
FOR
HOT
FLUSHES

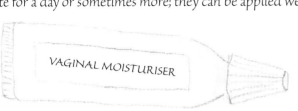

VAGINAL MOISTURISER

Over-The-Counter Alternatives

Phytoestrogens are compounds which have a weak oestrogen-like activity and are found in various whole grains, seeds, plants and beans. It has long been noted that women in Asia and Japan, whose diets are rich in phytoestrogens, experience far fewer menopausal symptoms, especially hot flushes, and have a lower incidence of osteoporosis. Further research is needed but many women find relief in supplementing their diet with these naturally occurring phytoestrogens.

Caution Please~ Phytoestrogens may be contraindicated for women with hormone dependant breast cancers because of their oestrogen-like activity. So anyone with a history of breast cancer, or other hormone dependant tumours, should always talk to their doctor about the safety of alternative therapies.

DANGER

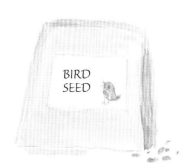

BIRD
SEED

Foods Rich In Phytoestrogens Include...

EAT YOUR GREENS...

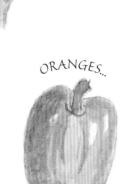

YOUR DAILY BREAD

WHOLE GRAIN CEREAL

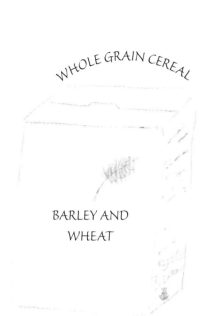

BARLEY AND
WHEAT

ORANGES...

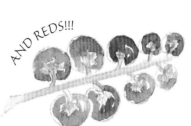

LEGUMES

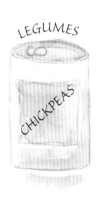

CHICKPEAS

AND REDS!!!

Red clover, soya and linseed oils contain a rich source of phytoestrogens. Soya and linseed can now be found in many products on the supermarket shelves, notably bread. Red clover can be bought in tablet form.

CAN BLACK COHOSH MAKE YOU FEEL LESS BLUE...

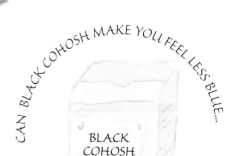

BLACK
COHOSH

Herbal remedies can also play a part in relieving menopausal symptoms. Although there is little scientific evidence for their effectiveness, many women use them and report benefits, including improvement in hot flushes, sweats and mood swings.

Helpful Herbs?

Agnus Castus ~ Upside ~ Generally balances hormones and helps with hot flushes.
Downsides ~ May interfere with contraceptives and HRT.

Sage ~ Upside ~ may help reduce hot flushes and night sweats.
Downside ~ may interact with blood pressure medication and tamoxifen.

Ginkgo Biloba ~ Upside~ may help improve memory
Downside ~ hard to remember how to spell it! More importantly, it should not be taken with warfarin or aspirin as it could increase risk of bleeding.

Black Cohosh ~ Upside ~ seems to help with mood swings and depression.
Downside ~ may interfere with blood pressure medication and may also cause a reaction in women who are allergic to aspirin.

Other Supplements Which Can Help Include...

Evening primrose oil and Starflower oil. They both contain an essential fatty acid, are commonly used for breast pain and tenderness and may also help with mood swings. But take care as both can interfere with epilepsy and blood pressure treatments.

Certain vitamins, especially C, B and E, are also on the honours list for helping women through the menopause.

READ THE LABEL

In Summary:

There are several prescribed and dozens of over-the-counter alternatives to HRT. There is very little scientific evidence to suggest that natural remedies work, but many women find benefit from some of these alternative therapies, which therefore gives them a rightful place on the shelves. But please remember before taking alternative remedies... READ THE LABEL and talk to your doctor, especially if you are on prescribed medication.

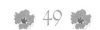

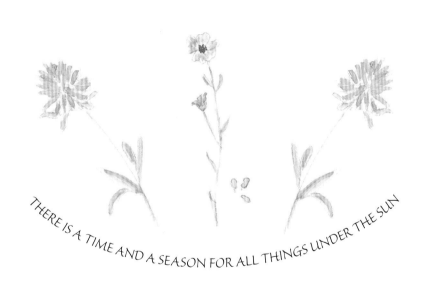

THERE IS A TIME AND A SEASON FOR ALL THINGS UNDER THE SUN

Chapter Nine

Keeping On Top Of Your Health

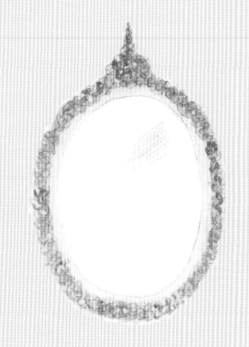

Time For A Check-Up

You may be susceptible, now or in the future, to a number of health issues, especially if you have a family history of medical problems. These can include heart disease, breast cancer, diabetes or a stroke, to name just a few. But help is at hand from both national screening programmes and from your own doctor.

It is advisable, with increasing age, to have your blood pressure, cholesterol and glucose (sugar) levels checked. Other tests may be required, depending on your past medical history, family history, any current medical problems or any medication you are on.

It is also important to discuss with your GP any irregular bleeding, especially that associated with abdominal pain or bleeding during or just after sex. A sudden onset of bleeding after the menopause also requires a trip to your doctor.

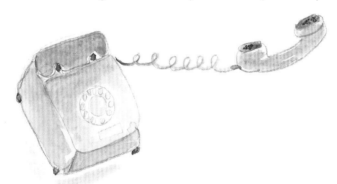

SOS

Screening programmes are an excellent way to check for any early signs of diseases. There are several such programmes in the UK, two of the most important being cervical smear tests and mammograms. Cervical smears screen to prevent cancer of the cervix and are routinely offered to women between the ages of 25-64, with routine recall every 3-5 years. Women between the ages of 50-70 are eligible for a mammogram to screen for any early signs of breast cancer. This is offered every three years and has been proven to be highly successful in the early diagnosis and treatment of breast cancer. Because of its success, it is hoped that the screening age range will be extended from 47-73 years of age in the near future.

So Take Up All That Is Offered To You...

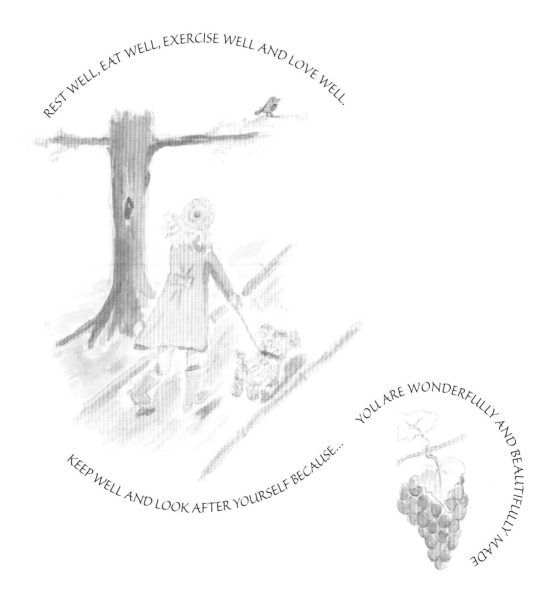

REST WELL, EAT WELL, EXERCISE WELL AND LOVE WELL.

KEEP WELL AND LOOK AFTER YOURSELF BECAUSE... YOU ARE WONDERFULLY AND BEAUTIFULLY MADE

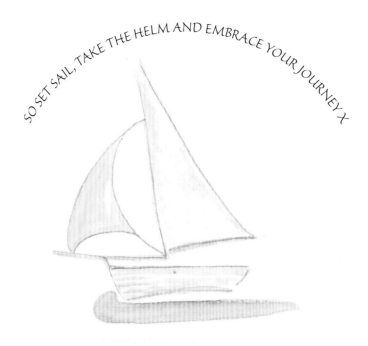

SO SET SAIL, TAKE THE HELM AND EMBRACE YOUR JOURNEY X

Glossary...

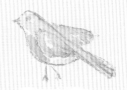

Amenorrhoea: the complete absence of any menstrual bleed.

BNF: British National Formulary. Found on almost every doctor's desk. A comprehensive guide on all prescribable medicines.

Caffeine: a stimulant found in drinks and some food. It may make hot flushes worse. Try decaf.

Climacteric: similar to the perimenopause. The changes that take place physically and emotionally around the menopause and the years leading up to it.

DEXA scan: Dual Energy X-ray Absorptiometry scan. A type of x-ray machine that measures bone mineral density. It is used in the diagnosis of osteoporosis .

Early menopause: a slightly arbitrary term but used when the menopause is diagnosed before the age of 45. See also premature menopause.

Endometriosis: a condition of unknown cause.

Cells from the endometrium (below) are found outside the womb and can grow in response to hormones. This can cause pain, especially with intercourse, ovarian cysts and infertility.

Endometrium: the lining of the womb.

FSH: Follicle Stimulating Hormone. Produced by the pituitary gland in the brain. It acts on the ovaries to help stimulate and mature eggs within follicles. It increases in concentration around the menopause and can be used to help diagnose the menopause.

HRT: Hormone Replacement Therapy. It does what it says on the label!

LH: Luteinising Hormone. Produced in the pituitary gland and acts on the ovary to trigger ovulation (release of an egg) around the mid-cycle.

Menopause: put simply, this is a woman's final menstrual period. The average age of the menopause in the UK is 51.

Oestrogen: a hormone produced by the ovaries. It is the decrease in concentration of this hormone that causes many of the symptoms experienced around the menopause.

Oophorectomy: the surgical removal of one or both ovaries.

Osteoporosis: a reduction in bone mineral density causing the skeleton to become more fragile.

Perimenopause: the time leading up to the menopause. Most commonly identified by irregular periods, hot flushes and emotional instability .

Phytoestrogens: compounds derived from plants that have oestrogen-like properties.

Postmenopause: the time of life after a woman's last ever menstrual bleed.

Premature Menopause: the term used when the menopause occurs before the age of 40. This can be naturally occurring or because of surgical removal of the ovaries. Chemotherapy can also cause a premature menopause. Unless treated, these younger women are at risk of heart disease, osteoporosis and possibly dementia.

Progesterone: a hormone produced by the ovaries that plays an essential role in the menstrual cycle. It also protects the womb lining (endometrium) from the risks of excess thickening or even womb cancer, that can be caused by oestrogen acting alone.

Progestogen: a synthetic form of progesterone. Several types are available.

SERMS: selective oestrogen receptor modulators. Synthetic drugs with oestrogen-like activity. They may be prescribed to help increase bone density and thereby reducing the risk of fractures, especially in the spine.

SSRIs: selective serotonin reuptake inhibitors. Commonly used as antidepressants, but can be helpful in reducing hot flushes and night sweats.

Time For Yourself: it speaks for itself and is essential.

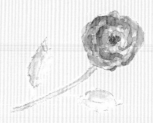

Addresses...

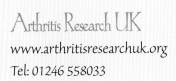
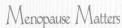

Arthritis Research UK
www.arthritisresearchuk.org
Tel: 01246 558033

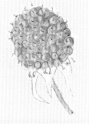

Cancer Advice
Offers specialist advice and support for cancer
patients and their families.
www.macmillan.org.uk
Tel: 020 7840 7840

Family Planning Association
Offers advice on sexual health
and contraception.
www.fpa.org.uk
Helpline: 0845 122 8690

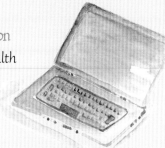

FRAX On-Line Questionnaire
www.Sheffield.ac.uk/FRAX
Assesses your risk of osteoporosis

Institute for Complementary Medicine
www.i-c-m.org.uk
Tel: 020 7922 7980

International Osteoporosis Foundation
www.iofbonehealth.org

Menopause Matters
An independent website and magazine led by specialists.
www.menopausematters.co.uk

National Institute For Health and Clinical Excellence (NICE)
www.nice.org.uk

National Osteoporosis Society
www.nos.org.uk
Helpline: 0845 450 0230

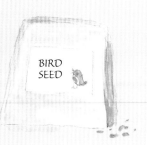

NHS Smoking Helpline
Freephone 0800 022 4332

Relate Marriage Guidance
Offers information on local approved Relate counsellors
www.relate.org.uk
Helpline: 0300 100 1234

The British Menopause Society
An excellent website on menopause health issues
www.thebms.org.uk

The Sixty Minute Marriage
An excellent short, wise and witty book on keeping your
relationship healthy.
Written by Rob Parsons
ISBN 0-340-67145-9

Index...

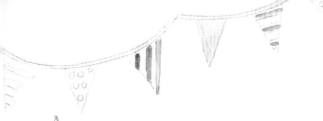

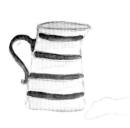

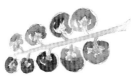
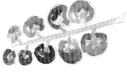
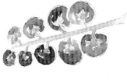

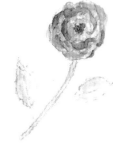
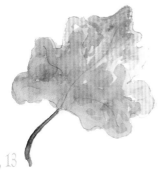
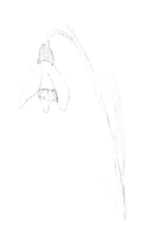

Your Notes...

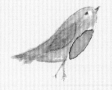

Your Notes...

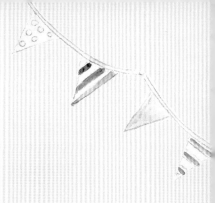

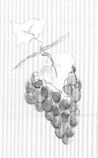

Your Notes...

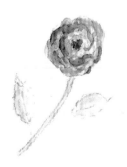

Your Notes...

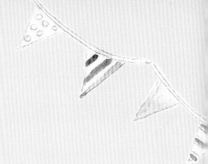

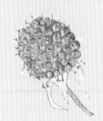

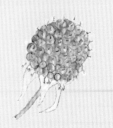

Your Notes...

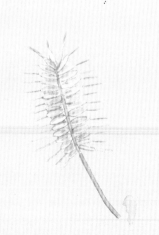

Your Notes...

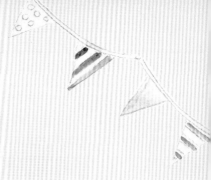

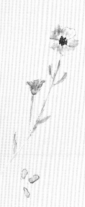

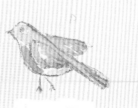

Keeping Your Cool In The
Heat Of The Night
A Survival Guide To The
Menopause

Published in the UK by Robin House Books
First Edition Published in 2011

Robin House Books
www.robinhousebooks.com
info@robinhousebooks.com

ISBN: 978-0-9569747-0-9

Printed and bound by The Five Castles Press Ltd, Ipswich, Suffolk

Written And Illustrated by Dr Louise Cowan
Design layout by Charlotte Cartwright

Robin House Books

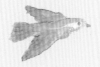

Dear Reader,
This book is intended as a guide to help you understand the menopause and it is not, in any way,
an alternative to seeking medical advice from your own doctor.
At the time of writing this book, the information contained within its pages is correct and current
to the best of my knowledge. Medicine rapidly evolves and so data, information and guidance can quickly
change or be updated.
Please ALWAYS discuss your health issues with your doctor and NEVER take any medication without first
consulting your doctor. Thank you, Dr Louise Cowan.